MW01275323

WFPB 90 Day Challenge

Whole Food Plant-Based Diet Journal & Food Log

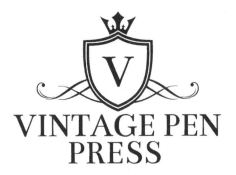

VINTAGE PEN PRESS

Thanks to EmojiOne for providing free emoji icons

Visit Us
www.vintagepenpress.com

~ INTRODUCTION ~

Are you ready to let plants rock your world? Take the next 90 days and increase the amount of fruits & vegetables in your diet - you'll be amazed with the results!

Use this food log and journal to track your daily servings of whole grains, beans & legumes, berries and other fruits, cruciferous vegetables, greens, nuts and seeds. Power Up your health with additional servings, track your hydration, and keep track of how you feel.

Look for ways to knock out a number of servings in one meal - like a large salad with greens, beans, fruit and nuts - BAM! Add hummus instead of mayo to a veggie sandwich and there's another serving of beans.

So what exactly is a serving? Great Question! Use the following guidelines to figure out servings for each category.

Whole Grains:
1/2 cup hot cereal or cooked grains, pasta, or corn kernels; 1 tortilla or slice of bread; 1 cup cold cereal; 3 cups popped popcorn; 1/2 a bagel or 1 English muffin

Beans:
1/4 cup hummus or bean dip; 1 cup of fresh peas or sprouted lentils; 1/2 cup cooked beans, split peas, lentils, tofu, or tempeh

Berries:
1/2 cup fresh or frozen; 1/4 cup dried

Other Fruits:
1 medium-sized fruit; 1 cup cut up fruit; 1/4 cup dried fruit

Greens:
1 cup raw; 1/2 cup cooked

Cruciferous Vegetables:
1/2 cup chopped; 1/4 cup brussels or broccoli sprouts; 1 tablespoon horseradish

Other Vegetables:
1 cup raw leafy vegetables; 1/2 cup raw or cooked non-leafy vegetables; 1/2 cup vegetable juice; 1/4 cup dried mushrooms

Flaxseed & Walnuts:
1 tablespoon flaxseed; 1/4 cup walnuts;

Other Nuts & Seeds:
1/4 cup nuts or seeds; 2 tablespoons nut or seed butter

"Let food be
thy medicine
and medicine
be thy food."
   - Hippocrates

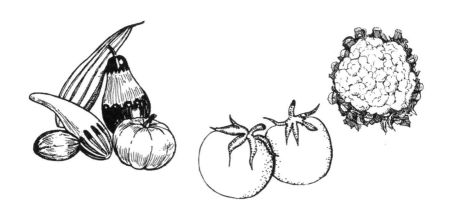

DATE: Jan 1/20

DAILY SERVINGS

POWER UP

- Whole Grains ☑☑☑☐ ✸
- Beans & Legumes ☑☐☐
- Berries ☐☐ ☆
- Other Fruits ☑☑
- Greens ☐☐ ☆
- Cruciferous Vegetables ☐ ☆
- Other Vegetables ☑ ☆
- Flaxseed & Walnuts ☐ ☆
- Other Nuts & Seeds ☑ Chia

KEEP HYDRATED:

TODAY I FEEL:

Oatmeal w Pears & cranberries + chia
                Banana
Jackfruit noodle soup + hummus sandwich
Taco chips, nuts n bolts, grapefruit
& 4 mini mandarins, chocolate
Started liquid calcium / magnesium

MY FAVORITE MEAL / RECIPE TODAY WAS...

Breakfast.

DATE: JAN 2/20

DAILY SERVINGS

POWER UP

		Servings	Power Up
🌾	Whole Grains	☑ ☑ ☐ ☐	☆
🫘	Beans & Legumes	☑ ☐ ☐	
🍓	Berries	☐ ☐	☆
🍐	Other Fruits	☑ ☑	
🥬	Greens	☐ ☐	☆
🥦	Cruciferous Vegetables	☐	☆
🌿	Other Vegetables	☐	☆
🌰	Flaxseed & Walnuts	☐	☆
🥜	Other Nuts & Seeds	☑	

KEEP HYDRATED:

TODAY I FEEL:

Oatmeal w pear / banana / cranberries
cooked in soy milk.
Same lunch as yesterday.
Chili & taco chips
Peanut brittle, chocolate

DID YOU KNOW?

Bell peppers are usually sold green, but they can also be
red, purple or yellow.

DATE: Jan 3/20

DAILY SERVINGS

POWER UP

- ✿ Whole Grains ☑ ☑ ☐ ☐ ☆
- ⚬ Beans & Legumes ☐ ☐ ☐
- 🍓 Berries ☐ ☐ ☆
- 🍐 Other Fruits ☐ ☐
- 🥬 Greens ☐ ☐ ☆
- 🥦 Cruciferous Vegetables ☐ ☆
- 🌱 Other Vegetables ☐ ☆
- 🌰 Flaxseed & Walnuts ☐ ☆
- 🥜 Other Nuts & Seeds ☑

KEEP HYDRATED:

TODAY I FEEL:

Griddler Hashbrowns
Set potatoes => preheat & sear @ 450

MY FAVORITE MEAL / RECIPE TODAY WAS...

Wednesday

DATE: Sept 23/20   DAILY SERVINGS   *POWER UP*

Whole Grains /spuds ☑☑☑☑ ☆

Beans & Legumes ☑☑☑

Berries ☑☑ ☆

Other Fruits ☑☑

Greens ☐☐ ☆

Cruciferous Vegetables ☑ ☆

Other Vegetables ☑ ☆

Flaxseed & Walnuts ☑ ☆

Other Nuts & Seeds ☐

KEEP HYDRATED:

TODAY I FEEL:

DID YOU KNOW?

Apples float in water because they are 25% air.

Thursday

DATE: Sept 24/20

DAILY SERVINGS

POWER UP

🌾 Whole Grains ☑ ☑ ☐ ☐ ☆

🫘 Beans & Legumes ☐ ☐ ☐

🍓 Berries ☑ ☑ ☆

🍐 Other Fruits ☑ ☐

🥦 Greens ☐ ☐ ☆

🥦 Cruciferous Vegetables ☑ ☆

🥕 Other Vegetables ☐ ☆

🌰 Flaxseed & Walnuts ☐ ☆

🥜 Other Nuts & Seeds ☐

KEEP HYDRATED:

TODAY I FEEL:

MY FAVORITE MEAL / RECIPE TODAY WAS...

DATE: _____

DAILY SERVINGS   *POWER UP*

Whole Grains   ☐ ☐ ☐ ☐   ☆
Beans & Legumes   ☐ ☐ ☐
Berries   ☐ ☐   ☆
Other Fruits   ☐ ☐
Greens   ☐ ☐   ☆
Cruciferous Vegetables ☐   ☆
Other Vegetables   ☐   ☆
Flaxseed & Walnuts   ☐   ☆
Other Nuts & Seeds   ☐

KEEP HYDRATED:

TODAY I FEEL:

_____

_____

_____

_____

_____

DID YOU KNOW?

Most of the nutrients in a potato reside just below the
skin layer.

DATE: _____   DAILY SERVINGS   *POWER UP*

🌾 Whole Grains ☐ ☐ ☐ ☐ ☆
🫘 Beans & Legumes ☐ ☐ ☐
🍓 Berries ☐ ☐ ☆
🍐 Other Fruits ☐ ☐
🥦 Greens ☐ ☐ ☆
🥦 Cruciferous Vegetables ☐ ☆
🥕 Other Vegetables ☐ ☆
🥜 Flaxseed & Walnuts ☐ ☆
🥜 Other Nuts & Seeds ☐

KEEP HYDRATED:

🥤 🥤 🥤 🥤 🥤 🥤

TODAY I FEEL:

🙂 😠 😆 🤒 😍 😴

_____

_____

_____

_____

_____

MY FAVORITE MEAL / RECIPE TODAY WAS...

_____

_____

_____

DATE: _____

DAILY SERVINGS

POWER UP

		Daily Servings	Power Up
🌾	Whole Grains	☐ ☐ ☐ ☐	☆
🫛	Beans & Legumes	☐ ☐ ☐	
🍓	Berries	☐ ☐	☆
🍐	Other Fruits	☐ ☐	
🥬	Greens	☐ ☐	☆
🥦	Cruciferous Vegetables	☐	☆
🌿	Other Vegetables	☐	☆
🌱	Flaxseed & Walnuts	☐	☆
🥜	Other Nuts & Seeds	☐	

KEEP HYDRATED:

TODAY I FEEL:

_____

_____

_____

_____

_____

DID YOU KNOW?

Ancient Greeks believed hazelnuts could treat coughing and baldness.

DATE: _____

DAILY SERVINGS   *POWER UP*

Whole Grains ☐ ☐ ☐ ☐   ☆

Beans & Legumes ☐ ☐ ☐

Berries ☐ ☐   ☆

Other Fruits ☐ ☐

Greens ☐ ☐   ☆

Cruciferous Vegetables ☐   ☆

Other Vegetables ☐   ☆

Flaxseed & Walnuts ☐   ☆

Other Nuts & Seeds ☐

KEEP HYDRATED:

TODAY I FEEL:

_____

_____

_____

_____

_____

MY FAVORITE MEAL / RECIPE TODAY WAS...

_____

_____

_____

DATE: _____

DAILY SERVINGS   *POWER UP*

🌾 Whole Grains   ☐ ☐ ☐ ☐   ☆
🐚 Beans & Legumes   ☐ ☐ ☐
🍓 Berries   ☐ ☐   ☆
🍐 Other Fruits   ☐ ☐
🥬 Greens   ☐ ☐   ☆
🥦 Cruciferous Vegetables ☐   ☆
🌱 Other Vegetables   ☐   ☆
🌿 Flaxseed & Walnuts ☐   ☆
🥜 Other Nuts & Seeds ☐

KEEP HYDRATED:

TODAY I FEEL:

_____

_____

_____

_____

_____

DID YOU KNOW?

Tomatoes are a fruit not a vegetable. Tomatoes are the
most popular fruits in the world.

DATE: _____

DAILY SERVINGS   *POWER UP*

🌾 Whole Grains ☐ ☐ ☐ ☐   ☆

🫘 Beans & Legumes ☐ ☐ ☐

🍓 Berries ☐ ☐   ☆

🍐 Other Fruits ☐ ☐

🥬 Greens ☐ ☐   ☆

🥦 Cruciferous Vegetables ☐   ☆

🥗 Other Vegetables ☐   ☆

🌰 Flaxseed & Walnuts ☐   ☆

〇 Other Nuts & Seeds ☐

KEEP HYDRATED:

🥤 🥤 🥤 🥤 🥤 🥤

TODAY I FEEL:

🙂 😠 😄 🤒 😍 😴

_____

_____

_____

_____

_____

MY FAVORITE MEAL / RECIPE TODAY WAS...

_____

_____

_____

DATE: _____

DAILY SERVINGS

POWER UP

- 🌾 Whole Grains   ☐ ☐ ☐ ☐   ☆
- 🫘 Beans & Legumes   ☐ ☐ ☐
- 🍓 Berries   ☐ ☐   ☆
- 🍐 Other Fruits   ☐ ☐
- 🥬 Greens   ☐ ☐   ☆
- 🥦 Cruciferous Vegetables   ☐   ☆
- 🥗 Other Vegetables   ☐   ☆
- 🌰 Flaxseed & Walnuts   ☐   ☆
- 🥜 Other Nuts & Seeds   ☐

KEEP HYDRATED:

🥛 🥛 🥛 🥛 🥛 🥛

TODAY I FEEL:

🙂 😠 😆 🤒 😍 😴

_____

_____

_____

_____

_____

DID YOU KNOW?

An average strawberry has around 200 seeds.

DATE: _____ DAILY SERVINGS *POWER UP*

🌾 Whole Grains ☐ ☐ ☐ ☐ ☆

🫘 Beans & Legumes ☐ ☐ ☐

🍓 Berries ☐ ☐ ☆

🍐 Other Fruits ☐ ☐

🥬 Greens ☐ ☐ ☆

🥦 Cruciferous Vegetables ☐ ☆

🥕 Other Vegetables ☐ ☆

🌰 Flaxseed & Walnuts ☐ ☆

🥜 Other Nuts & Seeds ☐

KEEP HYDRATED:

TODAY I FEEL:

_____

_____

_____

_____

_____

MY FAVORITE MEAL / RECIPE TODAY WAS...

_____

_____

_____

DATE: _____

DAILY SERVINGS

POWER UP

Whole Grains ☐ ☐ ☐ ☐ ☆

Beans & Legumes ☐ ☐ ☐

Berries ☐ ☐ ☆

Other Fruits ☐ ☐

Greens ☐ ☐ ☆

Cruciferous Vegetables ☐ ☆

Other Vegetables ☐ ☆

Flaxseed & Walnuts ☐ ☆

Other Nuts & Seeds ☐

KEEP HYDRATED:

TODAY I FEEL:

_____

_____

_____

_____

DID YOU KNOW?

A horn worm can eat an entire tomato plant by itself in one day!

DATE: _____

DAILY SERVINGS   *POWER UP*

🌾 Whole Grains   ☐ ☐ ☐ ☐   ☆
🫘 Beans & Legumes   ☐ ☐ ☐
🍓 Berries   ☐ ☐   ☆
🍐 Other Fruits   ☐ ☐
🥬 Greens   ☐ ☐   ☆
🥦 Cruciferous Vegetables ☐   ☆
🌱 Other Vegetables   ☐   ☆
🌰 Flaxseed & Walnuts   ☐   ☆
🥜 Other Nuts & Seeds   ☐

KEEP HYDRATED:

TODAY I FEEL:

_____

_____

_____

_____

_____

MY FAVORITE MEAL / RECIPE TODAY WAS...

_____

_____

_____

DATE: _____

DAILY SERVINGS

POWER UP

🌾 Whole Grains	☐ ☐ ☐ ☐	☆
🫘 Beans & Legumes	☐ ☐ ☐	
🍓 Berries	☐ ☐	☆
🍐 Other Fruits	☐ ☐	
🥬 Greens	☐ ☐	☆
🥦 Cruciferous Vegetables	☐	☆
🥕 Other Vegetables	☐	☆
🌰 Flaxseed & Walnuts	☐	☆
🥜 Other Nuts & Seeds	☐	

KEEP HYDRATED:

TODAY I FEEL:

_____

_____

_____

_____

_____

DID YOU KNOW?

Almonds can't grow on their own. They need bees to help them pollinate.

DATE: _____

DAILY SERVINGS   POWER UP

🌾 Whole Grains   ☐ ☐ ☐ ☐   ☆
🫘 Beans & Legumes   ☐ ☐ ☐
🍓 Berries   ☐ ☐   ☆
🍐 Other Fruits   ☐ ☐
🥬 Greens   ☐ ☐   ☆
🥦 Cruciferous Vegetables ☐   ☆
🌶 Other Vegetables   ☐   ☆
🥜 Flaxseed & Walnuts   ☐   ☆
🥚 Other Nuts & Seeds   ☐

KEEP HYDRATED:

TODAY I FEEL:

_____

_____

_____

_____

MY FAVORITE MEAL / RECIPE TODAY WAS...

_____

_____

DATE: _____

DAILY SERVINGS   *POWER UP*

		Servings	Power Up
🌾	Whole Grains	☐ ☐ ☐ ☐	☆
🫘	Beans & Legumes	☐ ☐ ☐	
🍓	Berries	☐ ☐	☆
🍎	Other Fruits	☐ ☐	
🥬	Greens	☐ ☐	☆
🥦	Cruciferous Vegetables	☐	☆
🥕	Other Vegetables	☐	☆
🌰	Flaxseed & Walnuts	☐	☆
🥜	Other Nuts & Seeds	☐	

KEEP HYDRATED:

TODAY I FEEL:

_____

_____

_____

_____

_____

DID YOU KNOW?

California produces almost all of the broccoli sold in the United States.

DATE:_____   DAILY SERVINGS   *POWER UP*

🌾 Whole Grains	☐ ☐ ☐ ☐	☆
🫘 Beans & Legumes	☐ ☐ ☐	
🍓 Berries	☐ ☐	☆
🍐 Other Fruits	☐ ☐	
🥬 Greens	☐ ☐	☆
🥦 Cruciferous Vegetables	☐	☆
🍆 Other Vegetables	☐	☆
🌰 Flaxseed & Walnuts	☐	☆
🥜 Other Nuts & Seeds	☐	

KEEP HYDRATED:

TODAY I FEEL:

_____

_____

_____

_____

_____

MY FAVORITE MEAL / RECIPE TODAY WAS...

_____

_____

_____

DATE: _____   DAILY SERVINGS   *POWER UP*

🌾 Whole Grains ☐☐☐☐ ☆
🫘 Beans & Legumes ☐☐☐
🍓 Berries ☐☐ ☆
🍐 Other Fruits ☐☐
🥬 Greens ☐☐ ☆
🥦 Cruciferous Vegetables ☐ ☆
🥗 Other Vegetables ☐ ☆
🌱 Flaxseed & Walnuts ☐ ☆
🥜 Other Nuts & Seeds ☐

KEEP HYDRATED:

TODAY I FEEL:

_____
_____
_____
_____
_____

DID YOU KNOW?

Dark green vegetables include more vitamin C than light
green color vegetables.

DATE: _____

DAILY SERVINGS   *POWER UP*

🌾 Whole Grains ☐ ☐ ☐ ☐   ☆

🫘 Beans & Legumes ☐ ☐ ☐

🍓 Berries ☐ ☐   ☆

🍐 Other Fruits ☐ ☐

🥬 Greens ☐ ☐   ☆

🥦 Cruciferous Vegetables ☐   ☆

🥗 Other Vegetables ☐   ☆

🌰 Flaxseed & Walnuts ☐   ☆

🥜 Other Nuts & Seeds ☐

KEEP HYDRATED:

🥛 🥛 🥛 🥛 🥛 🥛

TODAY I FEEL:

🙂 😠 😆 🤒 😍 😴

_____

_____

_____

_____

_____

MY FAVORITE MEAL / RECIPE TODAY WAS...

_____

_____

_____

DATE: _____

DAILY SERVINGS   *POWER UP*

🌾 Whole Grains   ☐ ☐ ☐ ☐   ☆
🫘 Beans & Legumes   ☐ ☐ ☐
🍓 Berries   ☐ ☐   ☆
🍐 Other Fruits   ☐ ☐
🥬 Greens   ☐ ☐   ☆
🥦 Cruciferous Vegetables ☐   ☆
🌱 Other Vegetables   ☐   ☆
🌰 Flaxseed & Walnuts   ☐   ☆
🥜 Other Nuts & Seeds   ☐

KEEP HYDRATED:

🥤 🥤 🥤 🥤 🥤 🥤

TODAY I FEEL:

🙂 😠 😆 🤒 😍 😴

_____

_____

_____

_____

_____

DID YOU KNOW?

White potatoes were first cultivated by local Indians in the Andes Mountains of South America.

DATE: _____

DAILY SERVINGS   *POWER UP*

🌾 Whole Grains	☐	☐	☐	☐
🫘 Beans & Legumes	☐	☐	☐	
🍓 Berries	☐	☐		
🍐 Other Fruits	☐	☐		
🥬 Greens	☐	☐		
🥦 Cruciferous Vegetables	☐			
🥕 Other Vegetables	☐			
🌿 Flaxseed & Walnuts	☐			
🥜 Other Nuts & Seeds	☐			

☆ (Whole Grains)
☆ (Berries)
☆ (Greens)
☆ (Cruciferous Vegetables)
☆ (Other Vegetables)
☆ (Flaxseed & Walnuts)

KEEP HYDRATED:

🥛 🥛 🥛 🥛 🥛 🥛

TODAY I FEEL:

🙂 😠 😆 🤒 😍 😴

_____

_____

_____

_____

MY FAVORITE MEAL / RECIPE TODAY WAS...

_____

_____

DATE: _____

DAILY SERVINGS

POWER UP

🌾 Whole Grains	☐ ☐ ☐ ☐	☆
🫘 Beans & Legumes	☐ ☐ ☐	
🍓 Berries	☐ ☐	☆
🍐 Other Fruits	☐ ☐	
🥬 Greens	☐ ☐	☆
🥦 Cruciferous Vegetables	☐	☆
🌱 Other Vegetables	☐	☆
🌿 Flaxseed & Walnuts	☐	☆
🥜 Other Nuts & Seeds	☐	

KEEP HYDRATED:

🥤 🥤 🥤 🥤 🥤 🥤

TODAY I FEEL:

🙂 😠 😂 🤒 🥰 😴

_____

_____

_____

_____

_____

_____

DID YOU KNOW?

Osage orange fruits are used to repel cockroaches.

DATE: _____

DAILY SERVINGS

POWER UP

Whole Grains ☐ ☐ ☐ ☐   ☆

Beans & Legumes ☐ ☐ ☐

Berries ☐ ☐   ☆

Other Fruits ☐ ☐

Greens ☐ ☐   ☆

Cruciferous Vegetables ☐   ☆

Other Vegetables ☐   ☆

Flaxseed & Walnuts ☐   ☆

Other Nuts & Seeds ☐

KEEP HYDRATED:

TODAY I FEEL:

_____

_____

_____

_____

_____

MY FAVORITE MEAL / RECIPE TODAY WAS...

_____

_____

_____

DATE: _____

DAILY SERVINGS

POWER UP

		Servings	Power Up
🌾	Whole Grains	☐ ☐ ☐ ☐	☆
🫘	Beans & Legumes	☐ ☐ ☐	
🍓	Berries	☐ ☐	☆
🍐	Other Fruits	☐ ☐	
🥬	Greens	☐ ☐	☆
🥦	Cruciferous Vegetables	☐	☆
🌶	Other Vegetables	☐	☆
🌰	Flaxseed & Walnuts	☐	☆
🥜	Other Nuts & Seeds	☐	

KEEP HYDRATED:

🥛 🥛 🥛 🥛 🥛 🥛

TODAY I FEEL:

🙂 😠 😆 🤒 😍 😴

_____

_____

_____

_____

_____

DID YOU KNOW?

Potatoes first appeared in Europe in 1586; they made it to North America in 1719.

DATE: _____

DAILY SERVINGS   POWER UP

🌾 Whole Grains ☐ ☐ ☐ ☐   ☆

🫘 Beans & Legumes ☐ ☐ ☐

🍓 Berries ☐ ☐   ☆

🍐 Other Fruits ☐ ☐

🥦 Greens ☐ ☐   ☆

🥦 Cruciferous Vegetables ☐   ☆

🍆 Other Vegetables ☐   ☆

🌰 Flaxseed & Walnuts ☐   ☆

🥜 Other Nuts & Seeds ☐

KEEP HYDRATED:

TODAY I FEEL:

_____

_____

_____

_____

MY FAVORITE MEAL / RECIPE TODAY WAS...

_____

_____

_____

DATE: _____

DAILY SERVINGS   *POWER UP*

🌾 Whole Grains	☐ ☐ ☐ ☐	☆
Beans & Legumes	☐ ☐ ☐	
🍓 Berries	☐ ☐	☆
Other Fruits	☐ ☐	
Greens	☐ ☐	☆
Cruciferous Vegetables	☐	☆
Other Vegetables	☐	☆
Flaxseed & Walnuts	☐	☆
Other Nuts & Seeds	☐	

KEEP HYDRATED:

🥛 🥛 🥛 🥛 🥛 🥛

TODAY I FEEL:

🙂 😠 😆 🤒 🥰 😴

_____

_____

_____

_____

_____

DID YOU KNOW?

Americans spend almost $800 million a year on peanut
butter and there are six cities in the US named Peanut.

DATE: _____   DAILY SERVINGS   POWER UP

🌾 Whole Grains　　　☐ ☐ ☐ ☐　　　☆

🫘 Beans & Legumes　☐ ☐ ☐

🍓 Berries　　　　　☐ ☐　　　　　☆

🍐 Other Fruits　　　☐ ☐

🥬 Greens　　　　　☐ ☐　　　　　☆

🥦 Cruciferous Vegetables　☐　　　☆

🥗 Other Vegetables　☐　　　　　　☆

🌰 Flaxseed & Walnuts　☐　　　　　☆

🥜 Other Nuts & Seeds　☐

KEEP HYDRATED:

🥛 🥛 🥛 🥛 🥛 🥛

TODAY I FEEL:

🙂 😠 😆 🤒 😍 😴

_____

_____

_____

_____

_____

MY FAVORITE MEAL / RECIPE TODAY WAS...

_____

_____

_____

DATE: _____   DAILY SERVINGS   *POWER UP*

- 🌾 Whole Grains ☐☐☐☐ ☆
- 🫘 Beans & Legumes ☐☐☐
- 🍓 Berries ☐☐ ☆
- 🍐 Other Fruits ☐☐
- 🥬 Greens ☐☐ ☆
- 🥦 Cruciferous Vegetables ☐ ☆
- 🥗 Other Vegetables ☐ ☆
- 🌿 Flaxseed & Walnuts ☐ ☆
- 🥜 Other Nuts & Seeds ☐

KEEP HYDRATED:

TODAY I FEEL:

_____

_____

_____

_____

_____

DID YOU KNOW?
An apple tree can produce up to 400 apples a year.

DATE: _____

DAILY SERVINGS

POWER UP

🌾 Whole Grains	☐ ☐ ☐ ☐	☆
🫘 Beans & Legumes	☐ ☐ ☐	
🍓 Berries	☐ ☐	☆
🍐 Other Fruits	☐ ☐	
🥬 Greens	☐ ☐	☆
🥦 Cruciferous Vegetables	☐	☆
🥕 Other Vegetables	☐	☆
🌰 Flaxseed & Walnuts	☐	☆
🥜 Other Nuts & Seeds	☐	

KEEP HYDRATED:

TODAY I FEEL:

_____

_____

_____

_____

_____

MY FAVORITE MEAL / RECIPE TODAY WAS...

_____

_____

_____

DATE: _____   DAILY SERVINGS   *POWER UP*

🌾 Whole Grains	☐ ☐ ☐ ☐	☆
🫘 Beans & Legumes	☐ ☐ ☐	
🍓 Berries	☐ ☐	☆
🍐 Other Fruits	☐ ☐	
🥬 Greens	☐ ☐	☆
🥦 Cruciferous Vegetables	☐	☆
🥕 Other Vegetables	☐	☆
🌿 Flaxseed & Walnuts	☐	☆
🥜 Other Nuts & Seeds	☐	

KEEP HYDRATED:

🥛 🥛 🥛 🥛 🥛 🥛

TODAY I FEEL:

🙂 😠 😄 🤒 😍 😴

_____

_____

_____

_____

_____

DID YOU KNOW?

Plums, peaches and pears are actually members of the
Rose family.

DATE: _____

DAILY SERVINGS   POWER UP

🌾 Whole Grains   ☐ ☐ ☐ ☐   ☆
🫘 Beans & Legumes   ☐ ☐ ☐
🍓 Berries   ☐ ☐   ☆
🍐 Other Fruits   ☐ ☐
🥬 Greens   ☐ ☐   ☆
🥦 Cruciferous Vegetables ☐   ☆
🌰 Other Vegetables   ☐   ☆
🌿 Flaxseed & Walnuts   ☐   ☆
🥜 Other Nuts & Seeds   ☐

KEEP HYDRATED:

TODAY I FEEL:

_____

_____

_____

_____

_____

MY FAVORITE MEAL / RECIPE TODAY WAS...

_____

_____

_____

DATE: _____   DAILY SERVINGS   *POWER UP*

🌾 Whole Grains	☐ ☐ ☐ ☐	☆
🫘 Beans & Legumes	☐ ☐ ☐	
🍓 Berries	☐ ☐	☆
🍐 Other Fruits	☐ ☐	
🥬 Greens	☐ ☐	☆
🥦 Cruciferous Vegetables	☐	☆
🍆 Other Vegetables	☐	☆
🌰 Flaxseed & Walnuts	☐	☆
🥜 Other Nuts & Seeds	☐	

KEEP HYDRATED:

☐ ☐ ☐ ☐ ☐ ☐

TODAY I FEEL:

🙂 😠 😄 🤒 😍 😴

_____

_____

_____

_____

_____

DID YOU KNOW?

40% of the world's almonds are bought by chocolate manufacturers.

DATE: _____   DAILY SERVINGS   *POWER UP*

Whole Grains ☐ ☐ ☐ ☐   ☆
Beans & Legumes ☐ ☐ ☐
Berries ☐ ☐   ☆
Other Fruits ☐ ☐
Greens ☐ ☐   ☆
Cruciferous Vegetables ☐   ☆
Other Vegetables ☐   ☆
Flaxseed & Walnuts ☐   ☆
Other Nuts & Seeds ☐

KEEP HYDRATED:

TODAY I FEEL:

_____

_____

_____

_____

_____

MY FAVORITE MEAL / RECIPE TODAY WAS...

_____

_____

_____

DATE: _____

DAILY SERVINGS   *POWER UP*

- Whole Grains ☐ ☐ ☐ ☐   ☆
- Beans & Legumes ☐ ☐ ☐
- Berries ☐ ☐   ☆
- Other Fruits ☐ ☐
- Greens ☐ ☐   ☆
- Cruciferous Vegetables ☐   ☆
- Other Vegetables ☐   ☆
- Flaxseed & Walnuts ☐   ☆
- Other Nuts & Seeds ☐

KEEP HYDRATED:

TODAY I FEEL:

_____

_____

_____

_____

DID YOU KNOW?

Strawberries and cashews are the only fruits that have their seeds on the outside unlike all other fruits which have their seeds inside.

DATE: _____

DAILY SERVINGS   POWER UP

🌾 Whole Grains   ☐ ☐ ☐ ☐   ☆

🫘 Beans & Legumes   ☐ ☐ ☐

🍓 Berries   ☐ ☐   ☆

🍐 Other Fruits   ☐ ☐

🥦 Greens   ☐ ☐   ☆

🥦 Cruciferous Vegetables ☐   ☆

🌶 Other Vegetables   ☐   ☆

🥜 Flaxseed & Walnuts   ☐   ☆

🥜 Other Nuts & Seeds   ☐

KEEP HYDRATED:

🥛 🥛 🥛 🥛 🥛 🥛

TODAY I FEEL:

😐 😠 😆 🤒 😍 😴

_____

_____

_____

_____

MY FAVORITE MEAL / RECIPE TODAY WAS...

_____

_____

_____

DATE: _____

DAILY SERVINGS   *POWER UP*

🌾 Whole Grains   ☐ ☐ ☐ ☐   ☆
🫘 Beans & Legumes   ☐ ☐ ☐
🍓 Berries   ☐ ☐   ☆
🍐 Other Fruits   ☐ ☐
🥬 Greens   ☐ ☐   ☆
🥦 Cruciferous Vegetables ☐   ☆
🌿 Other Vegetables   ☐   ☆
🌰 Flaxseed & Walnuts   ☐   ☆
🥜 Other Nuts & Seeds   ☐

KEEP HYDRATED:

TODAY I FEEL:

_____

_____

_____

_____

_____

DID YOU KNOW?

Kiwi contains twice as much Vitamin C as an orange.

DATE: _____

Whole Grains ☐ ☐ ☐ ☐ ☆

Beans & Legumes ☐ ☐ ☐

Berries ☐ ☐ ☆

Other Fruits ☐ ☐

Greens ☐ ☐ ☆

Cruciferous Vegetables ☐ ☆

Other Vegetables ☐ ☆

Flaxseed & Walnuts ☐ ☆

Other Nuts & Seeds ☐

KEEP HYDRATED:

TODAY I FEEL:

_____

_____

_____

_____

_____

MY FAVORITE MEAL / RECIPE TODAY WAS...

_____

_____

DATE: _____   DAILY SERVINGS   *POWER UP*

- 🌾 Whole Grains   ☐ ☐ ☐ ☐   ☆
- 🫘 Beans & Legumes   ☐ ☐ ☐
- 🍓 Berries   ☐ ☐   ☆
- 🍐 Other Fruits   ☐ ☐
- 🥬 Greens   ☐ ☐   ☆
- 🥦 Cruciferous Vegetables ☐   ☆
- 🌱 Other Vegetables   ☐   ☆
- 🌿 Flaxseed & Walnuts   ☐   ☆
- ⚇ Other Nuts & Seeds   ☐

KEEP HYDRATED:

🥤 🥤 🥤 🥤 🥤 🥤

TODAY I FEEL:

🙂 😠 😆 🤒 🥰 😴

_____

_____

_____

_____

_____

DID YOU KNOW?

In the 19th century British sailors ate limes to prevent Scurvy.

DATE: _____

DAILY SERVINGS   *POWER UP*

Whole Grains ☐ ☐ ☐ ☐   ☆

Beans & Legumes ☐ ☐ ☐

Berries ☐ ☐   ☆

Other Fruits ☐ ☐

Greens ☐ ☐   ☆

Cruciferous Vegetables ☐   ☆

Other Vegetables ☐   ☆

Flaxseed & Walnuts ☐   ☆

Other Nuts & Seeds ☐

KEEP HYDRATED:

TODAY I FEEL:

_____

_____

_____

_____

_____

MY FAVORITE MEAL / RECIPE TODAY WAS...

_____

_____

_____

DATE: _____

DAILY SERVINGS   *POWER UP*

🌾 Whole Grains   ☐ ☐ ☐ ☐   ☆
🫘 Beans & Legumes   ☐ ☐ ☐
🍓 Berries   ☐ ☐   ☆
🍐 Other Fruits   ☐ ☐
🥬 Greens   ☐ ☐   ☆
🥦 Cruciferous Vegetables ☐   ☆
🌱 Other Vegetables   ☐   ☆
🌰 Flaxseed & Walnuts   ☐   ☆
🥜 Other Nuts & Seeds   ☐

KEEP HYDRATED:

🥤 🥤 🥤 🥤 🥤 🥤

TODAY I FEEL:

😊 😠 😆 🤒 🥰 😴

_____

_____

_____

_____

_____

DID YOU KNOW?

There are over 7000 different types of apples grown all
over the world.

DATE: _____

DAILY SERVINGS   *POWER UP*

🌾 Whole Grains   ☐ ☐ ☐ ☐   ☆
🫘 Beans & Legumes   ☐ ☐ ☐
🍓 Berries   ☐ ☐   ☆
🍐 Other Fruits   ☐ ☐
🥬 Greens   ☐ ☐   ☆
🥦 Cruciferous Vegetables ☐   ☆
🫚 Other Vegetables   ☐   ☆
🌿 Flaxseed & Walnuts   ☐   ☆
🥜 Other Nuts & Seeds   ☐

KEEP HYDRATED:

🥛 🥛 🥛 🥛 🥛 🥛

TODAY I FEEL:

🙂 😠 😄 🤒 🥰 😴

_____

_____

_____

_____

_____

MY FAVORITE MEAL / RECIPE TODAY WAS...

_____

_____

_____

DATE: _____   DAILY SERVINGS   *POWER UP*

🌾 Whole Grains	☐ ☐ ☐ ☐	☆
🫘 Beans & Legumes	☐ ☐ ☐	
🍓 Berries	☐ ☐	☆
🍎 Other Fruits	☐ ☐	
🥬 Greens	☐ ☐	☆
🥦 Cruciferous Vegetables	☐	☆
🥗 Other Vegetables	☐	☆
🌰 Flaxseed & Walnuts	☐	☆
🥜 Other Nuts & Seeds	☐	

KEEP HYDRATED:

TODAY I FEEL:

_____

_____

_____

_____

_____

DID YOU KNOW?

You can speed up the ripening of a pineapple by standing
it upside down (on the leafy end).

DATE: _____

DAILY SERVINGS   *POWER UP*

- 🌾 Whole Grains ☐ ☐ ☐ ☐ ☆
- 🫘 Beans & Legumes ☐ ☐ ☐
- 🍓 Berries ☐ ☐ ☆
- 🍐 Other Fruits ☐ ☐
- 🥬 Greens ☐ ☐ ☆
- 🥦 Cruciferous Vegetables ☐ ☆
- 🥕 Other Vegetables ☐ ☆
- 🌰 Flaxseed & Walnuts ☐ ☆
- 🥜 Other Nuts & Seeds ☐

KEEP HYDRATED:

TODAY I FEEL:

_____

_____

_____

_____

MY FAVORITE MEAL / RECIPE TODAY WAS...

_____

_____

_____

DATE: _____

DAILY SERVINGS   *POWER UP*

Whole Grains ▢ ▢ ▢ ▢   ☆

Beans & Legumes ▢ ▢ ▢

Berries ▢ ▢   ☆

Other Fruits ▢ ▢

Greens ▢ ▢   ☆

Cruciferous Vegetables ▢   ☆

Other Vegetables ▢   ☆

Flaxseed & Walnuts ▢   ☆

Other Nuts & Seeds ▢

KEEP HYDRATED:

TODAY I FEEL:

_____

_____

_____

_____

_____

DID YOU KNOW?

You can make furniture with Pear wood (its hard).

DATE: _____

DAILY SERVINGS   *POWER UP*

- Whole Grains   ☐ ☐ ☐ ☐   ☆
- Beans & Legumes   ☐ ☐ ☐
- Berries   ☐ ☐   ☆
- Other Fruits   ☐ ☐
- Greens   ☐ ☐   ☆
- Cruciferous Vegetables   ☐   ☆
- Other Vegetables   ☐   ☆
- Flaxseed & Walnuts   ☐   ☆
- Other Nuts & Seeds   ☐

KEEP HYDRATED:

TODAY I FEEL:

_____

_____

_____

_____

_____

MY FAVORITE MEAL / RECIPE TODAY WAS...

_____

_____

_____

DATE: _____

DAILY SERVINGS

POWER UP

🌾 Whole Grains	☐ ☐ ☐ ☐	☆
🫘 Beans & Legumes	☐ ☐ ☐	
🍓 Berries	☐ ☐	☆
🍐 Other Fruits	☐ ☐	
🥬 Greens	☐ ☐	☆
🥦 Cruciferous Vegetables	☐	☆
🌱 Other Vegetables	☐	☆
🌰 Flaxseed & Walnuts	☐	☆
🥜 Other Nuts & Seeds	☐	

KEEP HYDRATED:

TODAY I FEEL:

_____

_____

_____

_____

_____

DID YOU KNOW?

There are over 200 different known species of raspberries but only 2 species are grown on a large scale.

DATE: _____   DAILY SERVINGS   *POWER UP*

🌾 Whole Grains	☐ ☐ ☐ ☐	☆
🫘 Beans & Legumes	☐ ☐ ☐	
🍓 Berries	☐ ☐	☆
🍐 Other Fruits	☐ ☐	
🥬 Greens	☐ ☐	☆
🥦 Cruciferous Vegetables	☐	☆
🥕 Other Vegetables	☐	☆
🌰 Flaxseed & Walnuts	☐	☆
🥜 Other Nuts & Seeds	☐	

KEEP HYDRATED:

TODAY I FEEL:

_____

_____

_____

_____

_____

MY FAVORITE MEAL / RECIPE TODAY WAS...

_____

_____

_____

DATE: _____   DAILY SERVINGS   *POWER UP*

🌾 Whole Grains	☐ ☐ ☐ ☐	☆
🫘 Beans & Legumes	☐ ☐ ☐	
🍓 Berries	☐ ☐	☆
🍎 Other Fruits	☐ ☐	
🥬 Greens	☐ ☐	☆
🥦 Cruciferous Vegetables	☐	☆
🥕 Other Vegetables	☐	☆
🌿 Flaxseed & Walnuts	☐	☆
🥜 Other Nuts & Seeds	☐	

KEEP HYDRATED:

🥤 🥤 🥤 🥤 🥤 🥤

TODAY I FEEL:

🙂 😠 😆 🤒 😍 😴

_____

_____

_____

_____

_____

DID YOU KNOW?

Macadamias have the hardest shell of any nut, taking 300
PSI of pressure to crack them open.

DATE: _____   DAILY SERVINGS   *POWER UP*

🌾 Whole Grains   ☐ ☐ ☐ ☐   ☆

🫘 Beans & Legumes   ☐ ☐ ☐

🍓 Berries   ☐ ☐   ☆

🍐 Other Fruits   ☐ ☐

🥬 Greens   ☐ ☐   ☆

🥦 Cruciferous Vegetables ☐   ☆

🎋 Other Vegetables   ☐   ☆

🌰 Flaxseed & Walnuts   ☐   ☆

🥜 Other Nuts & Seeds   ☐

KEEP HYDRATED:

🥤 🥤 🥤 🥤 🥤 🥤

TODAY I FEEL:

🙂 😠 😄 🤒 😍 😴

_____

_____

_____

_____

_____

MY FAVORITE MEAL / RECIPE TODAY WAS...

_____

_____

_____

DATE: _____   DAILY SERVINGS   *POWER UP*

🌾 Whole Grains   ☐ ☐ ☐ ☐   ☆
🫘 Beans & Legumes   ☐ ☐ ☐
🍓 Berries   ☐ ☐   ☆
🥑 Other Fruits   ☐ ☐
🥬 Greens   ☐ ☐   ☆
🥦 Cruciferous Vegetables ☐   ☆
🌿 Other Vegetables   ☐   ☆
🌰 Flaxseed & Walnuts   ☐   ☆
🥜 Other Nuts & Seeds   ☐

KEEP HYDRATED:

🥤 🥤 🥤 🥤 🥤 🥤

TODAY I FEEL:

🙂 😠 😄 🤒 😍 😴

_____

_____

_____

_____

_____

DID YOU KNOW?

There are seven varieties of avocados grown commercially in Texas, but the Hass is the most popular.

DATE: _____

DAILY SERVINGS

POWER UP

Whole Grains ☐ ☐ ☐ ☐ ☆

Beans & Legumes ☐ ☐ ☐

Berries ☐ ☐ ☆

Other Fruits ☐ ☐

Greens ☐ ☐ ☆

Cruciferous Vegetables ☐ ☆

Other Vegetables ☐ ☆

Flaxseed & Walnuts ☐ ☆

Other Nuts & Seeds ☐

KEEP HYDRATED:

TODAY I FEEL:

_____

_____

_____

_____

MY FAVORITE MEAL / RECIPE TODAY WAS...

_____

_____

DATE: _____

DAILY SERVINGS   *POWER UP*

🌾 Whole Grains	☐ ☐ ☐ ☐	☆
🫘 Beans & Legumes	☐ ☐ ☐	
🍓 Berries	☐ ☐	☆
🍐 Other Fruits	☐ ☐	
🥬 Greens	☐ ☐	☆
🥦 Cruciferous Vegetables	☐	☆
🍆 Other Vegetables	☐	☆
🌰 Flaxseed & Walnuts	☐	☆
🥜 Other Nuts & Seeds	☐	

KEEP HYDRATED:

🥛 🥛 🥛 🥛 🥛 🥛

TODAY I FEEL:

🙂 😠 😆 🤒 🥰 😴

_____

_____

_____

_____

_____

DID YOU KNOW?

Walnuts are the oldest known tree food - they date all the way back to 10,000 BC.

DATE:_____   DAILY SERVINGS   *POWER UP*

- 🌾 Whole Grains   ☐ ☐ ☐ ☐   ☆
- 🫘 Beans & Legumes   ☐ ☐ ☐
- 🍓 Berries   ☐ ☐   ☆
- 🍑 Other Fruits   ☐ ☐
- 🥬 Greens   ☐ ☐   ☆
- 🥦 Cruciferous Vegetables   ☐   ☆
- 🧅 Other Vegetables   ☐   ☆
- 🥜 Flaxseed & Walnuts   ☐   ☆
- 🥥 Other Nuts & Seeds   ☐

KEEP HYDRATED:

TODAY I FEEL:

_____

_____

_____

_____

_____

MY FAVORITE MEAL / RECIPE TODAY WAS...

_____

_____

_____

DATE: _____ DAILY SERVINGS *POWER UP*

🌾 Whole Grains ☐ ☐ ☐ ☐ ☆

🫘 Beans & Legumes ☐ ☐ ☐

🍓 Berries ☐ ☐ ☆

🍐 Other Fruits ☐ ☐

🥬 Greens ☐ ☐ ☆

🥦 Cruciferous Vegetables ☐ ☆

🍄 Other Vegetables ☐ ☆

🌿 Flaxseed & Walnuts ☐ ☆

🥜 Other Nuts & Seeds ☐

KEEP HYDRATED:

TODAY I FEEL:

_____

_____

_____

_____

DID YOU KNOW?

Grapefruit can actually react negatively with lots of drugs including cholesterol-lowering medications.

DATE: _____

DAILY SERVINGS   *POWER UP*

🌾 Whole Grains	☐ ☐ ☐ ☐	☆
🫘 Beans & Legumes	☐ ☐ ☐	
🍓 Berries	☐ ☐	☆
🍑 Other Fruits	☐ ☐	
🥬 Greens	☐ ☐	☆
🥦 Cruciferous Vegetables	☐	☆
🌱 Other Vegetables	☐	☆
🌿 Flaxseed & Walnuts	☐	☆
🥜 Other Nuts & Seeds	☐	

KEEP HYDRATED:

🥛 🥛 🥛 🥛 🥛 🥛

TODAY I FEEL:

🙂 😠 😄 🤒 😍 😴

_____

_____

_____

_____

_____

MY FAVORITE MEAL / RECIPE TODAY WAS...

_____

_____

_____

DATE: _____   DAILY SERVINGS   *POWER UP*

Whole Grains ☐ ☐ ☐ ☐   ☆

Beans & Legumes ☐ ☐ ☐

Berries ☐ ☐   ☆

Other Fruits ☐ ☐

Greens ☐ ☐   ☆

Cruciferous Vegetables ☐   ☆

Other Vegetables ☐   ☆

Flaxseed & Walnuts ☐   ☆

Other Nuts & Seeds ☐

KEEP HYDRATED:

TODAY I FEEL:

_____

_____

_____

_____

DID YOU KNOW?

Olive trees can live for more than 1000 years.

DATE: _____

DAILY SERVINGS   *POWER UP*

🌾 Whole Grains   ☐ ☐ ☐ ☐   ☆
🫘 Beans & Legumes   ☐ ☐ ☐
🍓 Berries   ☐ ☐   ☆
🍎 Other Fruits   ☐ ☐
🥬 Greens   ☐ ☐   ☆
🥦 Cruciferous Vegetables ☐   ☆
🎃 Other Vegetables   ☐   ☆
🌰 Flaxseed & Walnuts   ☐   ☆
🥜 Other Nuts & Seeds   ☐

KEEP HYDRATED:

🥤 🥤 🥤 🥤 🥤 🥤

TODAY I FEEL:

🙂 😠 😂 🤒 😍 😴

_____

_____

_____

_____

_____

MY FAVORITE MEAL / RECIPE TODAY WAS...

_____

_____

_____

DATE: _____   DAILY SERVINGS   *POWER UP*

Whole Grains ☐ ☐ ☐ ☐ ☆
Beans & Legumes ☐ ☐ ☐
Berries ☐ ☐ ☆
Other Fruits ☐ ☐
Greens ☐ ☐ ☆
Cruciferous Vegetables ☐ ☆
Other Vegetables ☐ ☆
Flaxseed & Walnuts ☐ ☆
Other Nuts & Seeds ☐

KEEP HYDRATED:

TODAY I FEEL:

_____

_____

_____

_____

_____

DID YOU KNOW?

Cranberries bounce when ripe.

DATE: _____

DAILY SERVINGS   *POWER UP*

Whole Grains ☐ ☐ ☐ ☐ ☆

Beans & Legumes ☐ ☐ ☐

Berries ☐ ☐ ☆

Other Fruits ☐ ☐

Greens ☐ ☐ ☆

Cruciferous Vegetables ☐ ☆

Other Vegetables ☐ ☆

Flaxseed & Walnuts ☐ ☆

Other Nuts & Seeds ☐

KEEP HYDRATED:

TODAY I FEEL:

_____

_____

_____

_____

_____

MY FAVORITE MEAL / RECIPE TODAY WAS...

_____

_____

DATE: _____

DAILY SERVINGS   *POWER UP*

🌾 Whole Grains   ☐ ☐ ☐ ☐   ☆
🫘 Beans & Legumes   ☐ ☐ ☐
🍓 Berries   ☐ ☐   ☆
🍐 Other Fruits   ☐ ☐
🥬 Greens   ☐ ☐   ☆
🥦 Cruciferous Vegetables ☐   ☆
🧄 Other Vegetables   ☐   ☆
🌰 Flaxseed & Walnuts ☐   ☆
🥜 Other Nuts & Seeds ☐

KEEP HYDRATED:

TODAY I FEEL:

_____
_____
_____
_____

DID YOU KNOW?

Texas adopted the pecan tree as its state tree in 1919.

DATE: _____

DAILY SERVINGS   *POWER UP*

🌾 Whole Grains	☐ ☐ ☐ ☐	☆
🫘 Beans & Legumes	☐ ☐ ☐	
🍓 Berries	☐ ☐	☆
🍐 Other Fruits	☐ ☐	
🥬 Greens	☐ ☐	☆
🥦 Cruciferous Vegetables	☐	☆
🎃 Other Vegetables	☐	☆
🌰 Flaxseed & Walnuts	☐	☆
🥜 Other Nuts & Seeds	☐	

KEEP HYDRATED:

🥛 🥛 🥛 🥛 🥛 🥛

TODAY I FEEL:

🙂 😠 😄 🤒 😍 😴

_____

_____

_____

_____

_____

MY FAVORITE MEAL / RECIPE TODAY WAS...

_____

_____

_____

DATE: _____   DAILY SERVINGS   *POWER UP*

🌾 Whole Grains ☐☐☐☐ ☆

🫘 Beans & Legumes ☐☐☐

🍓 Berries ☐☐ ☆

🍐 Other Fruits ☐☐

🥬 Greens ☐☐ ☆

🥦 Cruciferous Vegetables ☐ ☆

🌽 Other Vegetables ☐ ☆

🌰 Flaxseed & Walnuts ☐ ☆

🥜 Other Nuts & Seeds ☐

KEEP HYDRATED:

🥤 🥤 🥤 🥤 🥤 🥤

TODAY I FEEL:

🙂 😠 😄 🤒 😍 😴

_____

_____

_____

_____

_____

DID YOU KNOW?

A pineapple plant produces only one pineapple every 2 years.

DATE: _____   DAILY SERVINGS   *POWER UP*

Whole Grains   ☐ ☐ ☐ ☐   ☆

Beans & Legumes   ☐ ☐ ☐

Berries   ☐ ☐   ☆

Other Fruits   ☐ ☐

Greens   ☐ ☐   ☆

Cruciferous Vegetables   ☐   ☆

Other Vegetables   ☐   ☆

Flaxseed & Walnuts   ☐   ☆

Other Nuts & Seeds   ☐

KEEP HYDRATED:

TODAY I FEEL:

_____

_____

_____

_____

_____

MY FAVORITE MEAL / RECIPE TODAY WAS...

_____

_____

_____

DATE: _____   DAILY SERVINGS   *POWER UP*

🌾 Whole Grains ☐ ☐ ☐ ☐   ☆
🫘 Beans & Legumes ☐ ☐ ☐
🍓 Berries ☐ ☐   ☆
🍐 Other Fruits ☐ ☐
🥬 Greens ☐ ☐   ☆
🥦 Cruciferous Vegetables ☐   ☆
🌱 Other Vegetables ☐   ☆
🌿 Flaxseed & Walnuts ☐   ☆
🥜 Other Nuts & Seeds ☐

KEEP HYDRATED:

🥛 🥛 🥛 🥛 🥛 🥛

TODAY I FEEL:

🙂 😠 😄 🤒 🥰 😴

_____

_____

_____

_____

_____

DID YOU KNOW?

Japanese Yubari cantaloupes are the most expensive
fruit in the world; two melons once sold at auction for
$23,500.

DATE: _____

DAILY SERVINGS   *POWER UP*

🌾 Whole Grains   ☐ ☐ ☐ ☐   ☆
🫘 Beans & Legumes   ☐ ☐ ☐
🍓 Berries   ☐ ☐   ☆
🍐 Other Fruits   ☐ ☐
🥬 Greens   ☐ ☐   ☆
🥦 Cruciferous Vegetables ☐   ☆
🌱 Other Vegetables   ☐   ☆
🌰 Flaxseed & Walnuts   ☐   ☆
🥜 Other Nuts & Seeds   ☐

KEEP HYDRATED:

TODAY I FEEL:

_____

_____

_____

_____

_____

MY FAVORITE MEAL / RECIPE TODAY WAS...

_____

_____

_____

DATE: _____

| DAILY SERVINGS | POWER UP |

Whole Grains ☐ ☐ ☐ ☐ ☆
Beans & Legumes ☐ ☐ ☐
Berries ☐ ☐ ☆
Other Fruits ☐ ☐
Greens ☐ ☐ ☆
Cruciferous Vegetables ☐ ☆
Other Vegetables ☐ ☆
Flaxseed & Walnuts ☐ ☆
Other Nuts & Seeds ☐

KEEP HYDRATED:

TODAY I FEEL:

_____

_____

_____

_____

_____

DID YOU KNOW?

Before 2013, the biggest buyer of kale was Pizza Hut.
They used the kale as a garnish for their salad bars.

DATE: _____

DAILY SERVINGS   *POWER UP*

🌾 Whole Grains   ☐ ☐ ☐ ☐   ☆
🫘 Beans & Legumes   ☐ ☐ ☐
🍓 Berries   ☐ ☐   ☆
🍐 Other Fruits   ☐ ☐
🥬 Greens   ☐ ☐   ☆
🥦 Cruciferous Vegetables   ☐   ☆
🧅 Other Vegetables   ☐   ☆
🌰 Flaxseed & Walnuts   ☐   ☆
🥜 Other Nuts & Seeds   ☐

KEEP HYDRATED:

🥤 🥤 🥤 🥤 🥤 🥤

TODAY I FEEL:

🙂 😠 😄 🤒 😍 😴

_____

_____

_____

_____

_____

MY FAVORITE MEAL / RECIPE TODAY WAS...

_____

_____

_____

DATE: _____

DAILY SERVINGS

POWER UP

	Whole Grains	☐ ☐ ☐ ☐	☆
	Beans & Legumes	☐ ☐ ☐	
	Berries	☐ ☐	☆
	Other Fruits	☐ ☐	
	Greens	☐ ☐	☆
	Cruciferous Vegetables	☐	☆
	Other Vegetables	☐	☆
	Flaxseed & Walnuts	☐	☆
	Other Nuts & Seeds	☐	

KEEP HYDRATED:

TODAY I FEEL:

_____

_____

_____

_____

_____

DID YOU KNOW?

The Daikon radish can grow up to 3 feet long and weigh
up to 100 pounds!

DATE: _____   DAILY SERVINGS   *POWER UP*

🌾 Whole Grains	☐ ☐ ☐ ☐	☆
🫘 Beans & Legumes	☐ ☐ ☐	
🍓 Berries	☐ ☐	☆
🍎 Other Fruits	☐ ☐	
🥦 Greens	☐ ☐	☆
🥦 Cruciferous Vegetables	☐	☆
🥕 Other Vegetables	☐	☆
🌰 Flaxseed & Walnuts	☐	☆
🥜 Other Nuts & Seeds	☐	

KEEP HYDRATED:

🥤 🥤 🥤 🥤 🥤 🥤

TODAY I FEEL:

🙂 😠 😆 🤒 😍 😴

_____
_____
_____
_____
_____

MY FAVORITE MEAL / RECIPE TODAY WAS...

_____
_____
_____

DATE: _____   DAILY SERVINGS   *POWER UP*

🌾 Whole Grains ☐☐☐☐ ☆

🫘 Beans & Legumes ☐☐☐

🍓 Berries ☐☐ ☆

🍑 Other Fruits ☐☐

🥬 Greens ☐☐ ☆

🥦 Cruciferous Vegetables ☐ ☆

🍆 Other Vegetables ☐ ☆

🌰 Flaxseed & Walnuts ☐ ☆

🥜 Other Nuts & Seeds ☐

KEEP HYDRATED:

🥛 🥛 🥛 🥛 🥛 🥛

TODAY I FEEL:

🙂 😠 😄 🤒 🥰 😴

_____

_____

_____

_____

_____

DID YOU KNOW?

The inside of a cucumber can be 20 degrees cooler than the outside air.

DATE: _____

DAILY SERVINGS   *POWER UP*

🌾 Whole Grains   ☐ ☐ ☐ ☐   ☆

🫘 Beans & Legumes   ☐ ☐ ☐

🍓 Berries   ☐ ☐   ☆

🍐 Other Fruits   ☐ ☐

🥬 Greens   ☐ ☐   ☆

🥦 Cruciferous Vegetables ☐   ☆

🌰 Other Vegetables   ☐   ☆

🌿 Flaxseed & Walnuts   ☐   ☆

🥜 Other Nuts & Seeds   ☐

KEEP HYDRATED:

TODAY I FEEL:

_____

_____

_____

_____

_____

MY FAVORITE MEAL / RECIPE TODAY WAS...

_____

_____

_____

DATE: _____

DAILY SERVINGS

POWER UP

🌾 Whole Grains	☐ ☐ ☐ ☐	☆
🫘 Beans & Legumes	☐ ☐ ☐	
🍓 Berries	☐ ☐	☆
🍐 Other Fruits	☐ ☐	
🥬 Greens	☐ ☐	☆
🥦 Cruciferous Vegetables	☐	☆
🥗 Other Vegetables	☐	☆
🌰 Flaxseed & Walnuts	☐	☆
🥜 Other Nuts & Seeds	☐	

KEEP HYDRATED:

TODAY I FEEL:

_____

_____

_____

_____

_____

DID YOU KNOW?

Salgam sayu, meaning 'turnip juice', is a popular drink in Turkey - it has a dark red color, and is made of pickled purple or black carrots and flavored with the juice of fermented turnips.

DATE: _____

DAILY SERVINGS

POWER UP

🌾 Whole Grains	☐ ☐ ☐ ☐	☆
🫘 Beans & Legumes	☐ ☐ ☐	
🍓 Berries	☐ ☐	☆
🍑 Other Fruits	☐ ☐	
🥬 Greens	☐ ☐	☆
🥦 Cruciferous Vegetables	☐	☆
🌶 Other Vegetables	☐	☆
🌰 Flaxseed & Walnuts	☐	☆
🥜 Other Nuts & Seeds	☐	

KEEP HYDRATED:

TODAY I FEEL:

_____

_____

_____

_____

_____

MY FAVORITE MEAL / RECIPE TODAY WAS...

_____

_____

_____

DATE: _____   DAILY SERVINGS   *POWER UP*

🌾 Whole Grains ☐ ☐ ☐ ☐   ☆
🫘 Beans & Legumes ☐ ☐ ☐
🍓 Berries ☐ ☐   ☆
🍐 Other Fruits ☐ ☐
🥬 Greens ☐ ☐   ☆
🥦 Cruciferous Vegetables ☐   ☆
🫙 Other Vegetables ☐   ☆
🌿 Flaxseed & Walnuts ☐   ☆
🥜 Other Nuts & Seeds ☐

KEEP HYDRATED:

TODAY I FEEL:

_____

_____

_____

_____

_____

DID YOU KNOW?

The eggplant was introduced in the United States by
Thomas Jefferson in 1806.

DATE: _____

DAILY SERVINGS

POWER UP

Whole Grains ☐ ☐ ☐ ☐ ☆

Beans & Legumes ☐ ☐ ☐

Berries ☐ ☐ ☆

Other Fruits ☐ ☐

Greens ☐ ☐ ☆

Cruciferous Vegetables ☐ ☆

Other Vegetables ☐ ☆

Flaxseed & Walnuts ☐ ☆

Other Nuts & Seeds ☐

KEEP HYDRATED:

TODAY I FEEL:

_____

_____

_____

_____

_____

MY FAVORITE MEAL / RECIPE TODAY WAS...

_____

_____

_____

DATE: _____   DAILY SERVINGS   *POWER UP*

🌾 Whole Grains   ☐ ☐ ☐ ☐   ☆

🫘 Beans & Legumes   ☐ ☐ ☐

🍓 Berries   ☐ ☐   ☆

🍐 Other Fruits   ☐ ☐

🥬 Greens   ☐ ☐   ☆

🥦 Cruciferous Vegetables   ☐   ☆

🥗 Other Vegetables   ☐   ☆

🌰 Flaxseed & Walnuts   ☐   ☆

🥜 Other Nuts & Seeds   ☐

KEEP HYDRATED:

TODAY I FEEL:

_____

_____

_____

_____

_____

DID YOU KNOW?

Arachibutyrophobia is the fear of peanut butter sticking to
the roof of your mouth.

DATE: _____

DAILY SERVINGS   *POWER UP*

🌾 Whole Grains   ☐ ☐ ☐ ☐   ☆
🫘 Beans & Legumes   ☐ ☐ ☐
🍓 Berries   ☐ ☐   ☆
🍎 Other Fruits   ☐ ☐
🥦 Greens   ☐ ☐   ☆
🥦 Cruciferous Vegetables ☐   ☆
🌿 Other Vegetables   ☐   ☆
🥜 Flaxseed & Walnuts   ☐   ☆
🥜 Other Nuts & Seeds   ☐

KEEP HYDRATED:

🥤 🥤 🥤 🥤 🥤 🥤

TODAY I FEEL:

🙂 😠 😄 🤒 😍 😴

_____

_____

_____

_____

_____

MY FAVORITE MEAL / RECIPE TODAY WAS...

_____

_____

_____

DATE: _____

DAILY SERVINGS   *POWER UP*

🌾 Whole Grains   ☐ ☐ ☐ ☐   ☆
🫘 Beans & Legumes   ☐ ☐ ☐
🍓 Berries   ☐ ☐   ☆
🍐 Other Fruits   ☐ ☐
🥬 Greens   ☐ ☐   ☆
🥦 Cruciferous Vegetables ☐   ☆
🌱 Other Vegetables   ☐   ☆
🌿 Flaxseed & Walnuts   ☐   ☆
🥜 Other Nuts & Seeds   ☐

KEEP HYDRATED:

🥛 🥛 🥛 🥛 🥛 🥛

TODAY I FEEL:

🙂 😠 😄 🤒 😍 😴

_____

_____

_____

_____

_____

DID YOU KNOW?

Brazil nuts require a specific bee to be pollinated and
take as long as 10 to 30 years to mature.

DATE: _____

DAILY SERVINGS   *POWER UP*

🌾 Whole Grains ☐ ☐ ☐ ☐   ☆

🫘 Beans & Legumes ☐ ☐ ☐

🍓 Berries ☐ ☐   ☆

🍐 Other Fruits ☐ ☐

🥬 Greens ☐ ☐   ☆

🥦 Cruciferous Vegetables ☐   ☆

🥕 Other Vegetables ☐   ☆

🌰 Flaxseed & Walnuts ☐   ☆

🥜 Other Nuts & Seeds ☐

KEEP HYDRATED:

TODAY I FEEL:

_____

_____

_____

_____

_____

MY FAVORITE MEAL / RECIPE TODAY WAS...

_____

_____

_____

DATE: _____

		DAILY SERVINGS	*POWER UP*

Whole Grains ☐ ☐ ☐ ☐ ☆

Beans & Legumes ☐ ☐ ☐

Berries ☐ ☐ ☆

Other Fruits ☐ ☐

Greens ☐ ☐ ☆

Cruciferous Vegetables ☐ ☆

Other Vegetables ☐ ☆

Flaxseed & Walnuts ☐ ☆

Other Nuts & Seeds ☐

KEEP HYDRATED:

TODAY I FEEL:

_____

_____

_____

_____

_____

DID YOU KNOW?

Grown in Egypt since at least 2780 B.C., radishes were originally black

DATE: _____

DAILY SERVINGS

POWER UP

🌾 Whole Grains ☐ ☐ ☐ ☐ ☆

🫘 Beans & Legumes ☐ ☐ ☐

🍓 Berries ☐ ☐ ☆

🍐 Other Fruits ☐ ☐

🥬 Greens ☐ ☐ ☆

🥦 Cruciferous Vegetables ☐ ☆

🌱 Other Vegetables ☐ ☆

🌿 Flaxseed & Walnuts ☐ ☆

🥜 Other Nuts & Seeds ☐

KEEP HYDRATED:

TODAY I FEEL:

_____

_____

_____

_____

_____

MY FAVORITE MEAL / RECIPE TODAY WAS...

_____

_____

_____

DATE: _____

DAILY SERVINGS	POWER UP

🌾 Whole Grains ☐ ☐ ☐ ☐   ⭐

🫘 Beans & Legumes ☐ ☐ ☐

🍓 Berries ☐ ☐   ⭐

🍐 Other Fruits ☐ ☐

🥬 Greens ☐ ☐   ⭐

🥦 Cruciferous Vegetables ☐   ⭐

🍆 Other Vegetables ☐   ⭐

🌰 Flaxseed & Walnuts ☐   ⭐

🥜 Other Nuts & Seeds ☐

KEEP HYDRATED:

🥤 🥤 🥤 🥤 🥤 🥤

TODAY I FEEL:

🙂 😠 😄 🤒 🥰 😴

_____

_____

_____

_____

_____

DID YOU KNOW?

Lima beans are sometimes referred to as butter beans
because of their buttery texture and have been grown
and harvested in Peru for about seven thousand years.

DATE: _____

DAILY SERVINGS

POWER UP

🌾 Whole Grains	☐ ☐ ☐ ☐ ☆
🫘 Beans & Legumes	☐ ☐ ☐
🍓 Berries	☐ ☐ ☆
🍐 Other Fruits	☐ ☐
🥬 Greens	☐ ☐ ☆
🥦 Cruciferous Vegetables	☐ ☆
🍆 Other Vegetables	☐ ☆
🌰 Flaxseed & Walnuts	☐ ☆
🥜 Other Nuts & Seeds	☐

KEEP HYDRATED:

☐ ☐ ☐ ☐ ☐ ☐

TODAY I FEEL:

🙂 😠 😄 🤒 🥰 😴

_____

_____

_____

_____

_____

MY FAVORITE MEAL / RECIPE TODAY WAS...

_____

_____

_____

DATE: _____ DAILY SERVINGS *POWER UP*

🌾 Whole Grains	☐ ☐ ☐ ☐	☆
🫘 Beans & Legumes	☐ ☐ ☐	
🍓 Berries	☐ ☐	☆
🍎 Other Fruits	☐ ☐	
🥬 Greens	☐ ☐	☆
🥦 Cruciferous Vegetables	☐	☆
🥗 Other Vegetables	☐	☆
🌰 Flaxseed & Walnuts	☐	☆
🥜 Other Nuts & Seeds	☐	

KEEP HYDRATED:

🥤 🥤 🥤 🥤 🥤 🥤

TODAY I FEEL:

🙂 😠 😆 🤒 😍 😴

_____

_____

_____

_____

_____

DID YOU KNOW?

The humble radish is mentioned in numerous literary
works, including works by Sir Francis Bacon, Mark Twain
and Alexandere Dumas.

DATE: _____

DAILY SERVINGS   *POWER UP*

Whole Grains	☐ ☐ ☐ ☐	☆
Beans & Legumes	☐ ☐ ☐	
Berries	☐ ☐	☆
Other Fruits	☐ ☐	
Greens	☐ ☐	☆
Cruciferous Vegetables	☐	☆
Other Vegetables	☐	☆
Flaxseed & Walnuts	☐	☆
Other Nuts & Seeds	☐	

KEEP HYDRATED:

TODAY I FEEL:

_____

_____

_____

_____

_____

MY FAVORITE MEAL / RECIPE TODAY WAS...

_____

_____

_____

DATE: _____   DAILY SERVINGS   *POWER UP*

🌾 Whole Grains   ☐ ☐ ☐ ☐   ☆
🫘 Beans & Legumes   ☐ ☐ ☐
🍓 Berries   ☐ ☐   ☆
🍐 Other Fruits   ☐ ☐
🥬 Greens   ☐ ☐   ☆
🥦 Cruciferous Vegetables ☐   ☆
🧅 Other Vegetables   ☐   ☆
🌰 Flaxseed & Walnuts   ☐   ☆
🥜 Other Nuts & Seeds   ☐

KEEP HYDRATED:

🥤 🥤 🥤 🥤 🥤 🥤

TODAY I FEEL:

🙂 😠 😄 🤒 🥰 😴

_____

_____

_____

_____

_____

DID YOU KNOW?

Before the introduction of pumpkins to Europe, rutabagas
were carved to make lanterns to defend households from
evil spirits on All Hallows' Eve.

DATE: _____

DAILY SERVINGS

POWER UP

🌾 Whole Grains ☐ ☐ ☐ ☐ ☆

🫘 Beans & Legumes ☐ ☐ ☐

🍓 Berries ☐ ☐ ☆

🍐 Other Fruits ☐ ☐

🥬 Greens ☐ ☐ ☆

🥦 Cruciferous Vegetables ☐ ☆

🥗 Other Vegetables ☐ ☆

🌿 Flaxseed & Walnuts ☐ ☆

🥜 Other Nuts & Seeds ☐

KEEP HYDRATED:

TODAY I FEEL:

_____

_____

_____

_____

_____

MY FAVORITE MEAL / RECIPE TODAY WAS...

_____

_____

_____

DATE: _____   DAILY SERVINGS   *POWER UP*

🌾 Whole Grains   ☐ ☐ ☐ ☐   ☆
🫘 Beans & Legumes   ☐ ☐ ☐
🍓 Berries   ☐ ☐   ☆
🍐 Other Fruits   ☐ ☐
🥬 Greens   ☐ ☐   ☆
🥦 Cruciferous Vegetables   ☐   ☆
🧅 Other Vegetables   ☐   ☆
🌿 Flaxseed & Walnuts   ☐   ☆
🥜 Other Nuts & Seeds   ☐

KEEP HYDRATED:

TODAY I FEEL:

_____

_____

_____

_____

_____

DID YOU KNOW?

The fear of vegetables is called Lachanophobia.

~ CONGRATULATIONS~

You just rocked your 90 day whole foods plant based challenge!

If you enjoyed this challenge and log book, we'd love to hear from you. You can leave us a review on Amazon and hopefully inspire a few other people to give the challenge a try.

We'd also love to have you join us in our Facebook group at https://www.facebook.com/groups/vintagepenpress/

And of course, feel free to visit us any time at our website where you can see all our products and join our insider group to know about new releases, coupons and events.

www.vintagepenpress.com

NICOLE COLLET PCOS DIET
(LOW GLYCEMIC)

BREAKFAST

½ C GLUTEN-FREE OATS (QUICK)

1 TSP ZERO-CAL SWEETENER

½ C MIXED BERRIES   + CINNAMON

1 TBSP PEANUT BUTTER

SNACK

APPLE + ¼ C NUTS (PEANUTS) SHE USED
~~BANANA~~
OR
GRANOLA BAR

LUNCH

TUNA SANDWICHES

½ CAN WATER PACKED TUNA   ~~OR~~ EXTRA LEAN Deli meats. 2 slc

1 TBSP MAYO (GET CAL-REDUCED)

+ PICKLES + GREEN ONION

2 SLICES WHOLE GRAIN BREAD   + MUSTARD

1 C RAW VEGGIES — CARROTS, CELERY, CUCUMBER
+
2 TBSP HUMMUS OR 1 TBSP LIGHT DRESSING

SNACK

1 SERVING WHOLE GRAIN CRACKERS

1.5 OZ LIGHT CHEESE + CUCUMBERS
OR 1 SERVING

Made in the USA
San Bernardino, CA
02 December 2019

DINNER

1 C RICE / 1 C COOKED VEGGIES / 3 OZ CHICKEN BREAST

2 TSP LIGHT MARG.

2 C GREENS (OR 1C RAW VEGG 1C GRE
+ 1 TBSP LIGHT DRESSING